Paleo for Beginners-A Complete Guide

How the Paleo Diet Can Improve Your Life

By: Dana Whyte

PUBLISHERS NOTES

Disclaimer

This publication is intended to provide helpful and informative material. It is not intended to diagnose, treat, cure, or prevent any health problem or condition, nor is intended to replace the advice of a physician. No action should be taken solely on the contents of this book. Always consult your physician or qualified health-care professional on any matters regarding your health and before adopting any suggestions in this book or drawing inferences from it.

The author and publisher specifically disclaim all responsibility for any liability, loss or risk, personal or otherwise, which is incurred as a consequence, directly or indirectly, from the use or application of any contents of this book.

Any and all product names referenced within this book are the trademarks of their respective owners. None of these owners have sponsored, authorized, endorsed, or approved this book.

Always read all information provided by the manufacturers' product labels before using their products. The author and publisher are not responsible for claims made by manufacturers.

Paperback Edition

Manufactured in the United States of America

DEDICATION

This book is dedicated to my grandmother June and all other who have been eating Paleo all of their life. Grandma June showed me how to eat healthy and be healthy.

TABLE OF CONTENTS

CHAPTER 1- PALEO THE RIGHT DIET

Our ancestors–and I'm not just talking our Paleolithic ancestors, as this applies through most of human history–didn't run marathons. Steady-state cardio, which is for an hour or more at a time at 65% or more of max heart rate, just was not the norm for the human race.

Good cardio health is great. There is plenty to say for a strong heart and being able to maintain a strenuous activity for long periods of time. However, steady state cardio is not necessarily the way we want to go to achieve this.

Low levels of aerobic activity for long periods of time are great. Walk, jog, hike, bike, swim, etc. at less than 65% of max heart rate. Imagine our ancestors walking through the forest or across the Savannah as they track an animal or gather food or move from one temporary home to another. Even throw on a weight vest or carry a small child with you to replicate bringing home the hunt or a basket of produce or packing the few personal items you owned.

Or, well, to replicate carrying a small child. They did that a lot too. Imagine our more recent ancestors spending twenty hours a week at their farming duties. This sort of low-intensity aerobic activity does wonders for the human body, as has been shown repeatedly.

Shorter bursts of high-intensity cardio, such as jump roping, HIIT (High Intensity Interval Training), sprints, a mile run, etc. at a higher heart rate are great too. Our ancestors did move fast, and could even move fast well, but they tended to do it in shorter bursts than we do. They didn't run over 20 miles in three hours or less. They ran to catch a meal, or to get away from a predator. They ran after their children, who weren't penned in as often as ours are. Go out to the closest sidewalk and sprint for fifty or a hundred yards as fast as you can (after warming up a bit of course). Imagine a lion or a bear or something else big, clawed, and toothed coming after you. You want to be able to outrun that thing over short distances. Or go run a mile occasionally. Learn to jump rope well enough to do a double-under. It's all great.

But if you're getting your heart rate up over 65% of your max, you don't want to keep the activity up for too long. Why is that? I mean, don't we go into a gym, see all those people who stay on the treadmill beating their time and distance scores from last week, going for an hour at a time? Don't personal trainers tell us we need more cardio if we didn't burn enough fat since the last time we had our measurements taken?

Yes, but that's not necessarily good for us to do on a regular basis. It is especially detrimental to women. Perhaps doing steady state cardio occasionally won't have a negative impact, and nothing is to say that you can't ever occasionally train for a 5K or half-marathon or something that requires a bit more steady state cardio, but to base your fitness off of running hard for an hour multiple days a week can have some less than encouraging side effects.

One is that it simply doesn't burn fat as well as many of us would like to think. The body wants to conserve its energy, and will down-regulate metabolism to inhibit fat burning as we run more. If our metabolism is down-regulated, we're also burning less fat throughout the rest of the day as well.

Running doesn't build a lot of muscle. Yes, it will certainly build some, there's no arguing with that after you just start running and find that your legs and even abs are sore. But it tones up only specific muscles needed for the motion you are doing, and no more. A lot of muscles get left out, and there is virtually no progress on the muscles that running does use once they've become accustomed to the activity. Too much cardio can also pull resources away from building muscle if you are doing weight lifting and other muscle-building activities, so running an hour after you've been in the weight room all the time is a little counter-intuitive. Doing steady-state cardio for select periods of time to lean out a little extra may make some sense, but making it part of your routine all the time does not.

Studies also have shown that a lot of stead state cardio also down-regulates production of the thyroid hormone T3, as well as its effectiveness and metabolism. This is made worse with caloric restriction, which often goes along with too much cardio. T3 is a primary regulator of metabolism in the body, and having too little and what is available being less effective slows down metabolism. You may be burning more energy, but now your body is using and losing less because of a slower metabolism. Your treadmill may say you've burned 600 calories by running for an hour, but you may be burning significantly less because your body is holding on to every ounce of energy it can.

T3 also influences fat-regulating hormones. Healthy levels of T3 improve fat regulation and fat burning, while lower levels inhibit these.

Think about it. When you're running constantly, and hard, your body senses it as a stressor, an energy waster, and emergency. This isn't just the brief spurt of energy we demand from our body when running from danger, this is a cortisol-raising, energy-sucking, what-in-the-world-is-going-on stressor. The body wants to conserve that energy for you in this stressful time when it thinks you're using too much or not getting enough, just like it will try to conserve energy if it is starving.

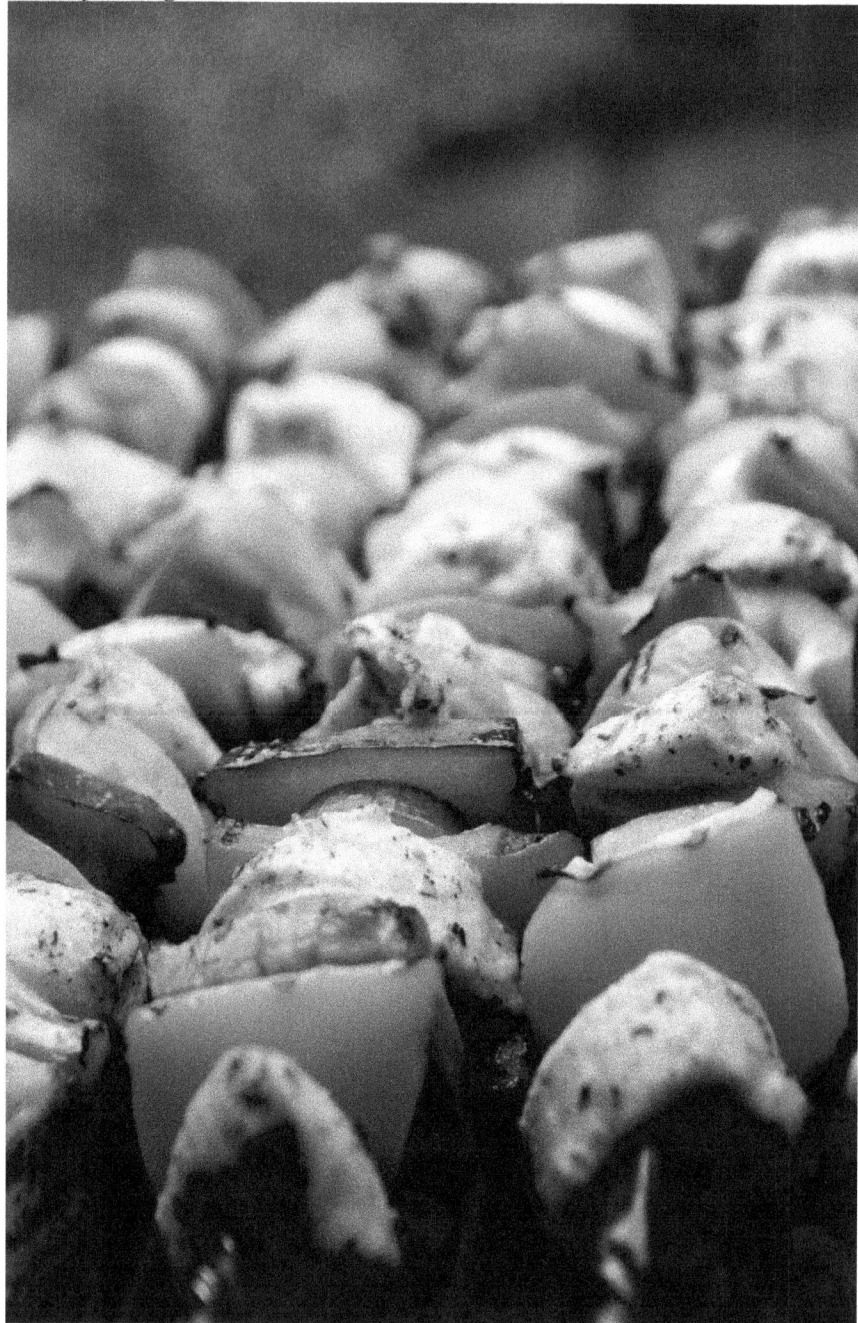

Doing sprints a couple of times a week won't do this to the body, as that just demands brief periods of extra energy that we probably have conserved and standing by if we're eating right. Taking long walks or hikes or a nicely paced bike ride won't do this to the body, as it simply tells the body that we are travelling or something else that our body is designed to do and which we can fuel well with a good diet. But we are taking the activity that we normally do when there is danger and excitement and adrenaline and we just. Keep. Doing. It. Over. And. Over. That's not giving your body good signals.

We are meant to be strong — to lift things up and put them down, especially if it's our own body. We are meant to be fast enough to catch dinner or to keep up with our own children as they play. We are meant to be able to move comfortably, often, steadily.

We are not meant to run from a lion for an hour or more. I promise, it will catch you by then.

Okay, okay, you say. You understand the concepts behind this, and that there are studies to back it up, and that HIIT-type training is becoming more popular because of all this. But I like running a 5K or even a marathon once or twice a year, you say.

That's fine. I am not here to say that you cannot pursue fitness your own way. And in fact, mixing in HIIT training can actually improve your steady-state performance. If you really want to run that race, or just like getting outside and pounding the pavement, then that's up to you. You should understand what it can potentially do to your body, and you should definitely make sure to do some strength training too. Be as good to your body as you can be if you're going to do regular steady-state cardio.

But if you've just been one of those people — particularly one of those women — who has been going into the gym and getting onto a treadmill for an hour because you think that's the best way for you to be skinny, fit, and healthy, then get off the dang treadmill and step into the weight room tomorrow. You will lose weight (unless you have more muscle to gain than fat to lose). Ladies, you won't bulk up but you'll certainly tone up. Men, you probably will bulk up a little, and most women really prefer a man who actually has biceps. You will be healthier. You will be stronger. And you'll probably like your body more

CHAPTER 2- OVERVIEW OF THE PALEO DIET – THE REAL TRUTH

A lot of people look at Paleo and think that it can't really be beneficial, it can't really help people lose weight. After all, it allows dark chocolate, wine, and bacon! This isn't a real diet!

First of all, Paleo is not a "diet" in the way many people normally think of diets. Normally the word "diet" evokes ideas of extreme restrictions, counting calories, rarely or never eating anything we really want, and even hunger and serious deprivation. We think of restriction diets. Paleo just doesn't fit into that paradigm, and for good reason.

Restriction diets don't work.

Yeah, maybe someone will lose weight on it initially, even be healthier. But restriction like that cannot be maintained, and when people break the diet, study after study shows that the weight comes back on. No one wants to feel hungry all the time. No one wants eating to be a chore. No one wants their dinner to depress them. No one wants to constantly be denied any and every tasty treat. These diets don't make permanent, sustainable change.

Some types of diets do tend to be more effective and sustainable than others. For instance, eating clean or Weight Watchers tend to get sustainable results. These are lifestyle diets which cut out or limit the worst types of foods and which allow a little bit of wiggle room. They have their downsides, but sustainable healthier eating and lifestyle changes work better than complete deprivation and restriction.

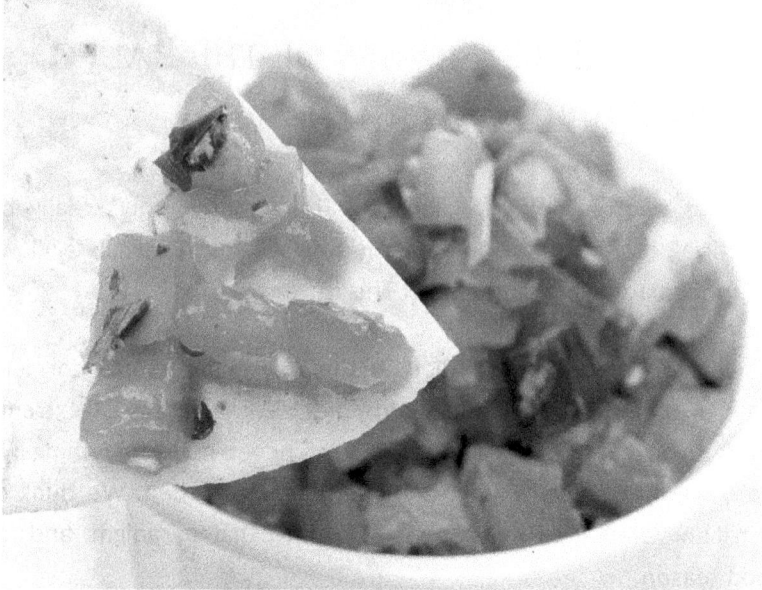

Paleo is a healthy change, a lifestyle diet that can be kept up indefinitely and even with enjoyment. It trumps even other lifestyle diets like clean eating, with its better macronutrient profile and food choices more natural to human diet and genetics. It kicks out gluten, unnecessary roughage, phytates, Omega-6 over-consumption, and excessive glucose. It increases nutrient intake, bumps up anti-oxidants, raises HDL, and works wonders on the GI tract.

Paleo isn't about restricting anything that we think might be bad for us. It's about pursuing health in a natural, big-picture sort of way.

Did you know dark chocolate has anti-oxidants? Yep, even better than many berries. It also has a great fat profile, improved arterial flow, lowers blood pressure, and can even make your skin more resistant to UV damage. And it really does ease PMS.

Did you know red wine contains resveratrol, which helps fight aging? Drinking it daily can also improve immunity to colds. Not to mention alcohol in moderation (no more than a few glasses a night) can help a person relax and de-stress.

Did you know bacon is well, just amazing? Eat it. Now. Really, it's just an animal product like any other meat, with wonderful fat and protein in it. A bit of extra sodium isn't so big of a deal on Paleo because you've cut out most sources already. Just be smart about where you get your bacon from.

It is far more important to have a sustainable diet with some wiggle room and the occasional treat allow than to deal with restriction, deprivation, and yo-yo dieting. We just make sure Paleo treats are smart, healthy, and, well, Paleo!

CAN YOU BECOME OVERWEIGHT ON THE PALEO DIET

There have been a couple of times now that I've been telling someone about Paleo and they're response is something along the lines of, "that's how I already eat!" And yet I look at them and they are severely overweight and unhealthy. How can someone who eats so healthily be so unhealthy?

The clues usually come quickly, as they reach for or share food or drink. They brought some baked good to the party that means they likely have white flour in their house. They pour a glass of sugar-laden juice as they share all about how they love this juice and chose it "because it had the least sugar!" as I stare at 32 grams on the nutrition label. They say no to the white bread but slather on the mayo. They happily reach for a mixed alcoholic beverage without even considering what's in it beyond the alcohol and taste.

They think they eat Paleo, or at least close to it, because Paleo makes sense to they and they know they should... but they really don't.

Paleo for Beginners

Are you one of those people? Do you even know if you're one of those people? Maybe you've thought you were eating Paleo, but your body is telling you (whether on the scale or some other way) that you're really not as healthy as you thought. Perhaps you have someone telling you they eat at least close to the Paleo guidelines, but you've seen them reach for something decidedly sub-standard enough times or have some other clue that makes you seriously doubt they're doing as well as they think they are.

If you're one of those people who isn't very sure, try keeping a food diary for a while. It may take no more than a day or two to realize that you're either writing in less-than-ideal food items, or that you're having to seriously think through what you reach for because what you would normally grab is something you don't want to have to write in.

Most people don't have to keep a food diary for more than a few weeks before they realize what changes to make and how they need to be made. If you find that keeping a food journal keeps you honest with yourself, then go ahead and keep writing it in, but don't feel like you have to once you've determined if you really are eating Paleo.

If you encounter someone who is asserting that they eat well but you have good reason to think they don't, it can be frustrating. Especially if they argue with you when you try to talk to them about it because they're so sure they're doing the right thing. You may not be able to help them out, and that's okay. It's their health, their fault, not yours.

But you can also use simple tools like asking them what they've eaten today, or what they ate yesterday, and telling them what isn't Paleo, or opening up their fridge and pointing out non-Paleo food items. Perhaps you can encourage them to do the food diary thing for their own awareness.

Dana Whyte

Many people are resistant to change, especially if they've convinced themselves they're doing well enough or like playing the unhealthy victim, but some people will be receptive once they realize that maybe they're not as healthy as they thought they were.

What matters most is your journey to health. Focus on yourself in this area. You can't help anyone else's health if you're neglecting your own, and convincing yourself that you're doing well enough if you're not is certainly not doing anything positive. Lead by example. If you can bring other people along as you get healthier, well, that's good too

CHAPTER 3- BLOOD TYPE OR CAVEMAN

A while back, I was encouraged by a coworker to check out the Eat Right for Your Type diet created and promoted by Dr D'Adamo. At first, I thought it sounded great. Both my husband and I are type A, so we would follow the same dietary guidelines. Perfect.

Then I actually took a closer look and did a little research, and it took all of about two links on a Google search to convince me that this diet was not what it was made out to be, and I abandoned it very quickly.

This diet is based on the idea that our blood types affect our digestion. This idea is this: O was the original blood type of our hunter-gatherer ancestors, and those with type O blood should continue to eat like that. But then types A, B, and AB come from varying agricultural societies, and those should eat more agrarian with limited meat and more grains and vegetables.

Type A supposedly flourishes on a vegetarian or near-vegetarian diet full of grains and produce. Type B was supposedly more nomadic and therefore should enjoy certain kinds of meat, plenty of dairy, and some produce but not grains. And type AB is somewhere in-between A and B, where they can enjoy more seafood but limit many other meats, can have dairy, and most produce.

D'Adamo claims this is because of lectins, which are food proteins that the different blood types react differently to. If this is true and our blood types handle certain foods better because of the compatibility with different lectins, then we should avoid the foods that have "harmful" lectins for our blood type. Using this idea, he gives each blood type a list of good foods, neutral foods, and bad foods for their type.

Dana Whyte

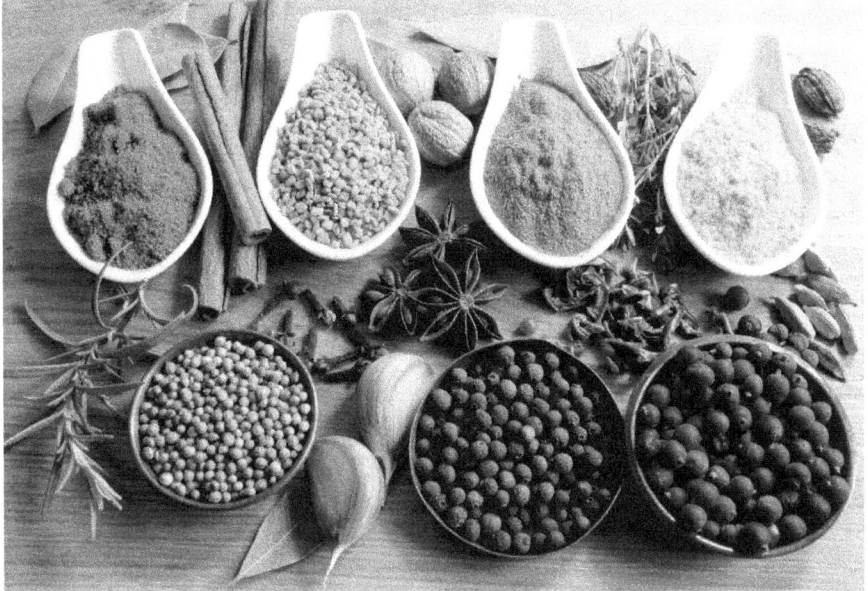

For many, this diet seems to work to at least some extent. I'd be interested to see if type O's, which are the most common blood type, tend to thrive off it most since they eat something similar to a Paleo, Atkins, or low-carb diet.

The diet in general lessens things like white flour, sugar, and preservatives even for type A, which means that someone who follows their blood type recommendations will likely be eating healthier than they were before and get at least some positive results. If you were eating donuts and nachos all the time before, and now you're eating lots of produce and grains are now whole, you're going to be healthier. It's a bit of a no-brainer.

On the other hand, the diet is neither ideal nor is the science supportable.

The research backing it up just isn't there. All D'Adamo has is anecdotal evidence, which can be explained by things much more supportable than lectins and blood types — my point above about the different diets causing generally healthier eating, for instance.

Further, his reasons for choosing each food type in the categories of beneficial, neutral, or avoid seems arbitrary and based on circular reasoning. He says type O should eat lots of meat because that's why type O originally ate, and so meat is good for people who are type O because that's what the blood type handles best. The evidence supporting each conclusion is lacking.

He also goes further in his book and recommends different natural remedies for diseases and illnesses based on blood type, but not one peer-reviewed article on PubMed in a search of his name reveals any support for his claims. While it is true that there are herbs and natural remedies that can help, perhaps significantly, which many ailments, the idea that it is based on blood type is completely unsupported and unsupportable.

The idea of lectins reacting specifically with different blood types is also unsupported by research. There are virtually no foods with ABO specific lectins, except just one or two like lima beans. Our everyday food certainly doesn't affect us based on our blood type.

It's hard to reasonably claim that our diet is affected by our blood type because of lectins when the lectins aren't blood-type specific.

The development of blood types proposed by D'Adamo is also under question. For instance, it's possible that type A was the original blood type rather than O. More importantly, no matter which blood type came first, our bodies cannot have changed so drastically based on blood type. There is limited genetic variation in the human population, and there has been very little genetic change compared to our Neolithic ancestors.

As if all that weren't enough, there is the evidence that supports what does affect our bodies and our weight in relation to diet, and it has far more to do with tested and tried things like insulin and carbohydrates. Lectins and blood types have nothing to do with a healthy, natural diet according to this research. Although conventional wisdom is still taking its time, kicking and screaming, to catch up to the research, the truth is there and it can be found.

I remember starting Paleo, and out of curiosity sitting down with D'Adamo's book *"Cook Right for Your Type."* I thumbed through the recipes, and surprise, surprise! I wasn't impressed by almost any of them. Only perhaps a handful in the type O were alright. There was way too much soy, legumes, dairy, and grain throughout.

This diet appeals to people because it seems more scientific, but unfortunately it's not. Only if you are type O will you potentially be eating at least close to ideally.

While people do tend to get healthier on this diet due to its promotion of healthier whole foods than they were probably eating before, it is not the truly ideal diet for the human body. That is has been peddled as scientific is a travesty.

CHAPTER 4- SLEEP AND PALEO HAND IN HAND

Diet and sleep are closely related, and all the good you're doing during the day can be harmed by not getting enough quality sleep. If you find yourself waking up groggy, shorting yourself on sleep, walking around with dark circles under your eyes, and all manner of indications of sleep deprivation, you need to fix it. Now.

Sleep is directly related to diet in that your body regulates hormones in your sleep, including those that regulate hunger and satiation signals. If you're shorting yourself on sleep, you'll feel hungrier and will overeat more easily.

The best diet can still be undone by stuffing yourself full of way too many calories. A body that is getting the correct signals at the correct times will usually regulate calorie intake much more effectively.

You also secrete human growth hormones while you sleep–which, by the way, makes kid's sleeping in the dark important to their growth. But this hormone doesn't only help kids; it helps you too, just not to grow taller. This hormone plays a role in cellular regeneration, which we all have need of.

Muscle repair, endocrine balancing, neurological functioning, mood, and your immune system are all impacted by sleep.

Don't think it's important yet?

Over time, sleep deprivation and harm long-term memory, generation of nerve cells, increase risk of mental illnesses and psychological disorders, and boost inflammation. Your heart and kidneys are impacted. Your blood pressure may go up. Your risk for obesity, diabetes, and other diseases increases.

You will actually die of sleep deprivation before you will die of starvation.

Yeah, it's really that serious.

Sleep deprivation also impacts cortisol levels negatively. Cortisol is normal for our body, but its release at the wrong times or in excessive amounts has an undesirable impact.

Normal release helps us wake up refreshed, and then declines through the day so that by bedtime so that other hormones release and we can get to sleep. If our sleep is sporadic or too short (and if we don't manage our stress levels, as chronic stress messes with cortisol), cortisol levels will be too high at night and may not release at the right time in the morning. And thus we have a nation of very tired people who can't get to sleep at night and have to drag themselves out of bed in the morning. No fun. Keep that up, and you'll get adrenal fatigue. Even more no fun.

So how do we go about reversing and improving these sleep related issues? Sleep!

First, how much sleep? Conventional wisdom is actually right on this one — 8 hours is enough for most people on average. It's not quite a magic number, however. Children need more. Elderly seem to need less, but really it's just broken up. Some adults can get by on 6-7, especially during young adulthood, and others function best on 9-10. It's been shown that mortality rates are higher both for those who routinely get 5 or less and for those who routinely get 11 or more. 7-9 is probably a reliable range.

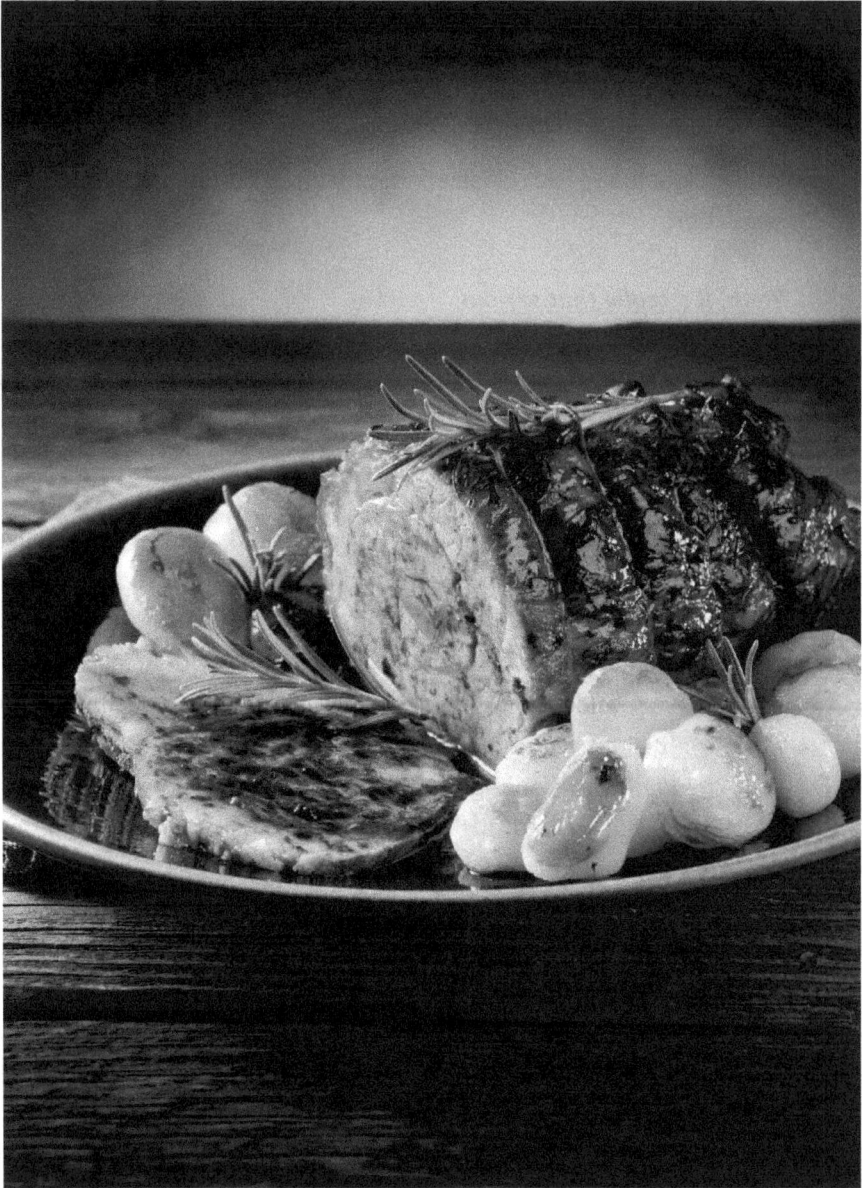

How does this sleep thing work? We go through a few stages of sleep. There are three stages of non-REM sleep called N1, N2, and N3. N1 is that light sleep where we can pull out easily and may even still be somewhat aware of our surroundings. From there it progresses through N2, which is basically a middle stage, and into the very deep sleep of N3, where people sleep through thunderstorms and puttering spouses. REM sleep then is where most (but not all) of our dreaming occurs, and we spend about a quarter of our sleep here.

Because of the phases, not all sleep is equal. If we're getting very broken sleep and therefore spending more time in the first couple of lighter-sleep, less restive stages, we won't get as much rest as if we get to go through enough deep and REM sleep stages.

Doing your best to make sure there are as few interruptions as possible, if any, is a good idea. Obviously a young couple can't stop their baby from waking up a few times through the night, but they may be able to make the interruptions as short and stress-free as possible.

Co-sleeping has actually been shown to help with this. You can also do things like turn on a fan so that little noises don't bother you (great for pet owners!).

Dark is also essential. More specifically, the exclusion of any blue, white, and violet lights. Think sunshine, computer screens, TV's, and fluorescents. The night colors are red, yellow, and orange.

Think firelight, red lamps, and perhaps certain types of light bulbs. An hour or more before bed, start transferring to light sources of the latter type. There is a program called flux for Windows that can change the color tone of a computer screen based on date, time, and your location.

It's best to sleep in pitch black. This helps your body with proper hormone regulation during sleep. And eye pillow isn't enough. Block out all light possible, especially lights of the daytime wavelengths mentioned above. Get solid curtains and close the blinds, especially if you sleep in a brightly lit area or in the daytime.

Turn out as many house lights as possible, and close the door if you need to. Put a yellow or red nightlight in the bathroom so you don't have to turn a big light on. Don't keep a TV in the bedroom, or make sure it's turned off a while before bedtime.

Establish a bedtime ritual, whether you have five minutes or an hour to put into it. Begin with transferring to the night-colored lights. Reading a book by candlelight, stretching, self-pampering, snuggle time with your spouse (or other types of time with your spouse), or other relaxation techniques are all good options. It should start you relaxing, help you de-stress, and eventually become a mental "it's time to go to sleep" signal.

Go to bed at about the same time every night. Yes, the occasional night out with friends, project at work, or upset child is going to get in the way of this habit. But if you can get close most of the time, your body will become used to it and even get back to it quickly after interruption. Your body will learn when to produce the sleepy hormones and reduce the wakeful hormones.

Wake up at about the same time daily. If you're getting enough sleep through the week, sleeping three extra hours Saturday morning isn't really necessary, so don't change your weekend schedule too much. If you do vary, get back on track the next day. When you go to bed, tell yourself your wake up time. You may find yourself no longer needing an alarm clock most of the time. What do you think they did before alarms, after all?

Dana Whyte

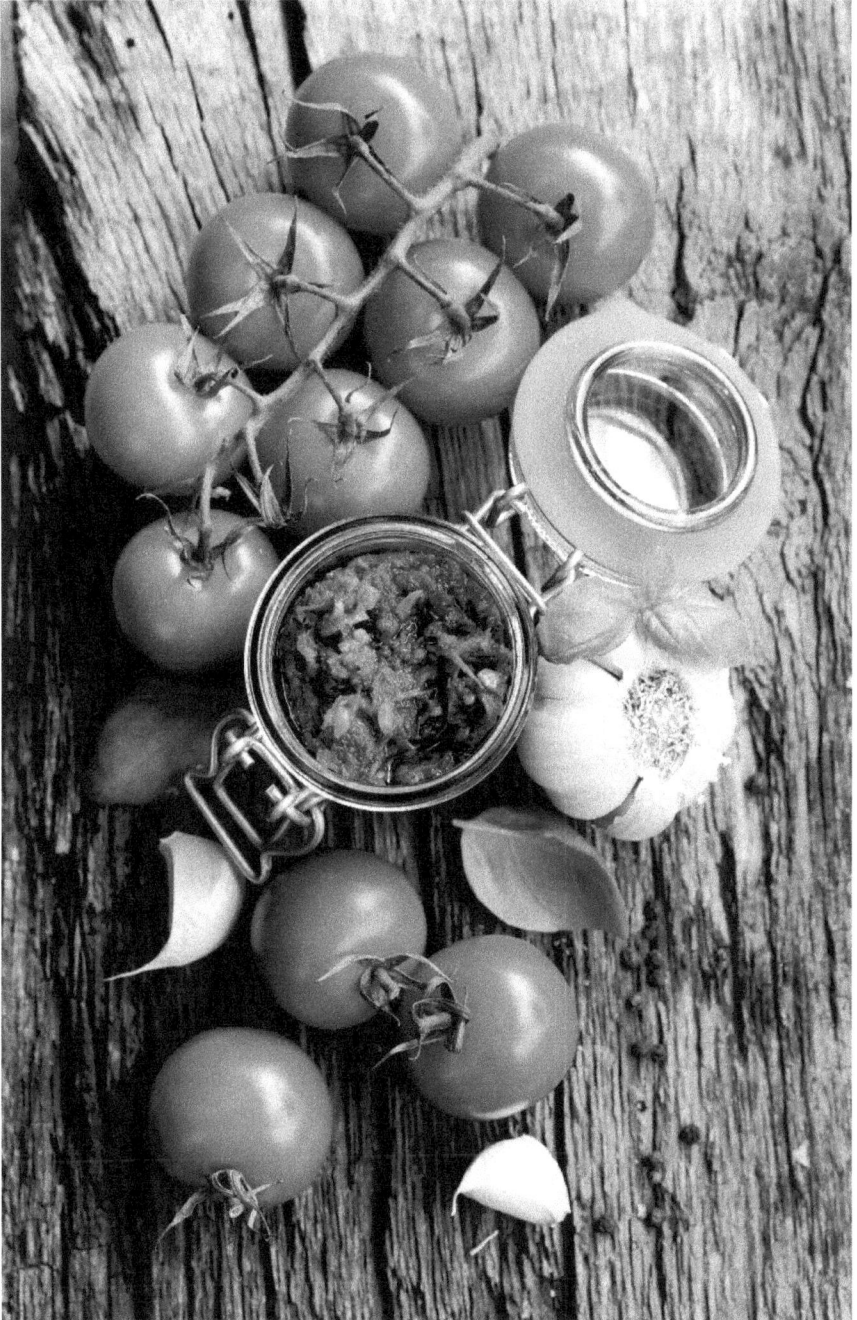

Naps are a viable option, although you want to try to get them long enough before bedtime that you won't be kept up because of it. Early afternoon is a great time. Hey moms, try napping when your kids do if you're short on sleep!

There will possibly be a rough period when you begin, particularly if your sleep schedule was all over the place or your sleep deprivation significant before. It takes a while for the body to put those hormones back in line. Just keep going. Your body will adjust eventually.

If your hormones are just too out of whack or you're exhausting yourself getting up on time after taking forever to get to sleep, some temporary melatonin supplementation may help. Use for the first day or two after changing shifts or getting to a new time zone would probably help as well, to mitigate "jet lag" and other schedule-change effects.

This should be used as a reset tool rather than as something to depend on. Extended use can cause the body to rely on the supplement rather than on producing its own, as the body will adjust its own output to account for input. Temporary use will act as a sort of signal for the body so that it can learn when it's supposed to be producing the hormone itself.

What's your bedtime ritual? What tricks did you use to improve quality of sleep? What helped you most if you have/had small children? What improvements did you see? Quicker muscle gain, improved immunity, better appetite control, more consistent and improved energy

Chapter 5- The 80% - 20%Rule Of Paleo Cooking

The idea of continuing 100% strict Paleo after your 30 day challenge might be pretty daunting, or just unrealistic. Perhaps you've found, through experimentation that the occasional sushi roll, glass of wine, bakes potato, or raw cheese is enjoyable and largely tolerable. Maybe your family likes doing a monthly get-together and they don't eat Paleo. In the least. Or you don't want to feel guilty if you eat this food, or have to be rude by rejecting it.

We totally get it, and we totally agree. Unless you have a severe intolerance to something, the stress and guilt of feeling you can't dish up Mom's signature dish or go out with friends is probably not worth it.

Here is where we come to the 80/20 rule. The idea is that you can get most of the benefits of Paleo by doing it 80% of the time, assuming you're not completely trashing it with the other 20%. A roll with dinner every night probably isn't going to fly, but a family dinner, an evening out with friends, communion at church, or a gray area food a few days a week aren't going to be your downfall.

Be smart about it. When you go to a restaurant, choose carefully. Maybe you should get that steak instead of Alfredo Maybe a salad instead of mozzarella sticks. Ask for the burger to be served without a bun. See if they have sweet potato fries instead of regular. Ask if they can cook your salmon in butter. Request their gluten-free options. Choose red win over a rum and Coke (I know, is blasphemy). Have them make a Paleo margarita. It takes some thought and planning — and maybe being a picky customer — but you can do it.

If you're being smart and careful, don't sweat the rest. Your 20% probably won't kill you, as long as your waiter doesn't. And while you should feel free to tell your family about Paleo, please don't insult the in-law's cooking.

ARE YOU ALLERGIC TO THE PALEO DIET

It's pretty easy to be skeptical about whether our bodies really don't like this stuff we've eaten all our lives, especially if we've never come up gluten or lactose intolerant. We're fine! Aren't we?

This is actually part of why we encourage people to do 30 strict days. If our bodies are used to "tolerating" something, we're not going to know how badly it will affect us if we continue asking our bodies to "tolerate" it. Only by letting our bodies adjust to being without something and then testing it again can we get an idea of how it really influences us.

Many times, our bodies will start readjusting in just a few days, but it will usually take two or more weeks to really make the change we're looking for. Some foods, like wheat, only need be ingested every couple of weeks to do damage and continue its vicious cycle in our bodies. That's not to say your 30 day challenge was useless if you have a cheat day, but you may not get the full effect.

After you've given your body a good acclimation period, add a food back in. Have some pasta with a baguette for dinner, for instance. You want to try each food a couple days apart. Your body probably hates grains, but may be okay with Greek yogurt sometimes, and you won't know which reacted badly if you add both back in the same day. You may also want to try different products within the same category on different days, as some are more offensive than others. The occasional bit of rice at your favorite Asian restaurant may be alright, but wheat may be the bane of your existence. That's pretty common, actually. A glass of pasteurized, homogenized milk may be your stomach's nightmare, but a bit of raw cheese may be nice occasionally. Only experimentation will tell.

Your body will be able to tell you what it doesn't like. You may feel symptoms as mild as simply a heavy, overly full stomach, or it may be much worse. Bloating, differences in bowel movements (particularly unpleasant differences), gas, cramping, indigestion, heartburn, lethargy, sugar highs and crashes, or a more vague feeling of sickness can all indicate problematic reactions to a food. Most or all grains, pasteurized milk, legumes, and sugar-filled foods will likely induce the worst reactions.

What' great about dairy self-experimentation is that it gives you qualitative evidence as to the effectiveness of Paleo and the reasons why these foods are less than optimal for human consumption. It's one thing to read about the ravages of gluten or undetected lactose sensitivity, it's a whole other thing to have your body tell you unequivocally that that means you!

So please, occasionally have that pizza and beer with the guys. Scarf that whole King Size Reese's package. Slather refried beans on a corn tortilla taco. It's nice to have a cheat day sometimes, and the intestinal Armageddon will remind you why you stopped eating that way in the first place. Then go tell your friends about the difference. In graphic detail. Anyone who's sat too long on the porcelain throne after some bean chili might think twice.

Let us know how your personal experiments go. What do you react worse to? What's okay? Is there anything you didn't even try to add in because you knew you'd react badly? Is there anything you're unusually sensitive to, like nightshades?

CHAPTER 6- DON'T GET SCAMMED

A couple of weeks back I saw a Facebook post about a diet called the liquid amino diet. There was a before and after picture of a woman who had lost a fair bit of weight on it, so I checked it out. I was quite unimpressed with what I found.

Basically, the diet called for "eating clean" and only getting about 1,000 calories a day. I wasn't able to find the specifics on the diet– they want you to buy a book. So already we're seeing weight loss through significant calorie deficit, and perhaps improved food choices, plus the requirement of shelling out money to know how to do it.

The second infuriating thing I found was the amino drops part of the diet. The formula is "exclusive" and a whopping $97 for a single bottle. Then I took a look at the ingredients in the "homeopathic" solution, and found some interesting things.

The first ingredient listed is phytolacca berry, and is actually poisonous raw. Another is graphite. As in, what's in pencils? Seriously? How do these things cause weight loss? Part of the idea of homeopathy is that "like cures like." As in, if you have a teeny tiny amount of something bad, it will make the bad go away.

But it's such a teeny tiny amount, that it really doesn't do much of anything to you. Perhaps this has a positive placebo-type effect for some people, but it's so medically unimportant that homeopathic medicines don't even have to go through testing–including testing to prove that it works.

$97 for something that doesn't work, and for a diet that does (sort of) work which you could do for free.

This bothers me profoundly, to tell the truth. This diet "works" through significant caloric restriction, but charges a ton of money for something else that doesn't work.

So many people are uninformed on how a healthy diet actually works, and don't realize that while many natural medical practices and herbs work, many like this are worthless and unproven in any real trials. People who don't understand these things are easily taken advantage of by people who want to make money off such lack of information instead of work to fix it.

Many effective plans have things that involve spending money. Books, cookbooks, supplements. If they work, if they teach, if they help, great. But good plans can and do also work for free–or for grocery costs, anyways. It's a scam to take advantage and charge exorbitant amounts for unnecessary products, especially if they don't work.

Moral of the story: be careful what you buy. You don't always get what you pay for.

Paleo for Beginners

CHAPTER 7- RECIPES WE LOVE!

Main Dishes and Casseroles

Super Simple Meatloaf

(_Serves 6_)

1 cup Stove Top Stuffing, crushed

2 cups canned spaghetti sauce with garlic and onions

1 1/2 lb. lean ground beef

Directions: Preheat oven to 350 degrees. Mix stuffing and 1 1/2 cups spaghetti sauce. (Save 1/2 cup sauce for later use.) Add ground beef to stuffing and sauce mix, and mix thoroughly. Spread mixture in loaf pan and cook uncovered for 1 hour. Spread remaining 1/2 cup sauce over loaf and cook for 30 minutes longer, or to desired doneness.

Category: Meat, Poultry and Seafood

Easy and Healthy Chicken Nuggets

(Serves 4)

1 lb. boneless, skinless chicken breast

3 egg whites

1 6oz. box Stove Top Stuffing

Dana Whyte

Directions: Preheat oven to 425 degrees. Cut chicken into bite-size pieces and trim off any fat. In bowl, beat egg whites for 30 seconds. Pour stuffing into heavy plastic bag and crush into crumbs using hammer or rolling pin. Pour crumbs into a bowl. Dip each piece of chicken into egg whites, then into crumbs. Coat heavily and place on cookie sheet that has been sprayed with nonstick cooking spray. Bake for 10 minutes, turn, and bake 10 minutes longer, or until crispy outside and cooked throughout.

Category: Pies, Pastries & Desserts

Cold Cantaloupe Summer Soup

(Serves 6)

1 cup orange juice

2 extra ripe, large cantaloupes

1/2 cup yogurt, any flavor

Directions: Peel cantaloupes and remove seeds. Chop into small pieces and place in blender. Add orange juice and yogurt, and puree just until well blended. Pour into mugs and freeze just until slushy.

So I kind of changed just about EVERYTHING but her recipe was my inspiration! The recipe really only had avocado, salt, and lime - no bacon and no cheese. For some reason I just felt the need to add the rest. I was glad I did. Allen didn't like the Asia go cheese so I used Colby Jack cheese - shredded...it was very tasty as well.

My Favorite Avocado Dish

1 HAAS Avocado

1 Lime - Juiced

2 Large Basil Leaves - Coarsely Chopped or Torn

Kosher Salt

Ground Black Pepper

1 Slice Bacon - Cooked & Crumbled

Asia go Cheese - Shredded

1 Large Slice Sourdough Bread

Butter

Direct

Combine avocado, lime juice, salt, pepper, and basil leaves.

Butter both sides of the bread and add to a skillet heated over medium heat until bread is crispy.

Layer bread, avocado spread, asiago cheese, and finally the bacon!!

This was so easy and the flavors were very good. Maybe next time though I will try it with powdered sugar instead of regular sugar - either way it will be one we make again!!

French My Toast

Dana Whyte

I substituted 2 teaspoons of vanilla extract for 2 teaspoons of orange liqueur, used half and half, sourdough bread and I did not put oil in the skillet.

(**We should not really eat bread on the Paleo Diet**)

2 Eggs

2 Teaspoons Vanilla Extract

2 Teaspoons Orange Liqueur

1/4 Cup Half & Half

2 Large Slices Sourdough Bread

2 Tablespoons Butter

Sugar

Maple Syrup

Whisk together eggs, vanilla, orange liqueur, and half and half. Pour into a 9X9 pan.

Lay bread slices in the egg mixture and soak for 5 minutes on each side.

Heat butter in a skillet over medium high heat and cook for 3-4 minutes on each side or until brown.

Remove from skillet and dredge slices in sugar. Drizzle with maple syrup.

I took the title of this recipe literally - EVOLUTION - I took his basic recipe and changed it to my liking. He added mint, olives, and red chills. I decided to try my own version and it was really very nice.

Cucu Mumber Salad

2 English Cucumbers - Peeled/Seeded/Cut into Large Chunks

1 Jalapeno - Seeded/Minced

1 Bundle Green Onions - Sliced

6 Tablespoon Extra Virgin Olive Oil

1 Lemon - Zest/Juiced

1 Heaping Tablespoon Low Fat Plain Yogurt

Kosher Salt

Ground Black Pepper

Combine cucumbers, jalapeno, and green onions in a medium size bowl.

Combine oil, zest, juice, and yogurt in a small bowl; whisk together all ingredients.

Toss together the veggies and dressing; season with salt and pepper. I would recommend letting this sit in the fridge for at least 4 hours to let the flavors work their magic together.

Dana Whyte

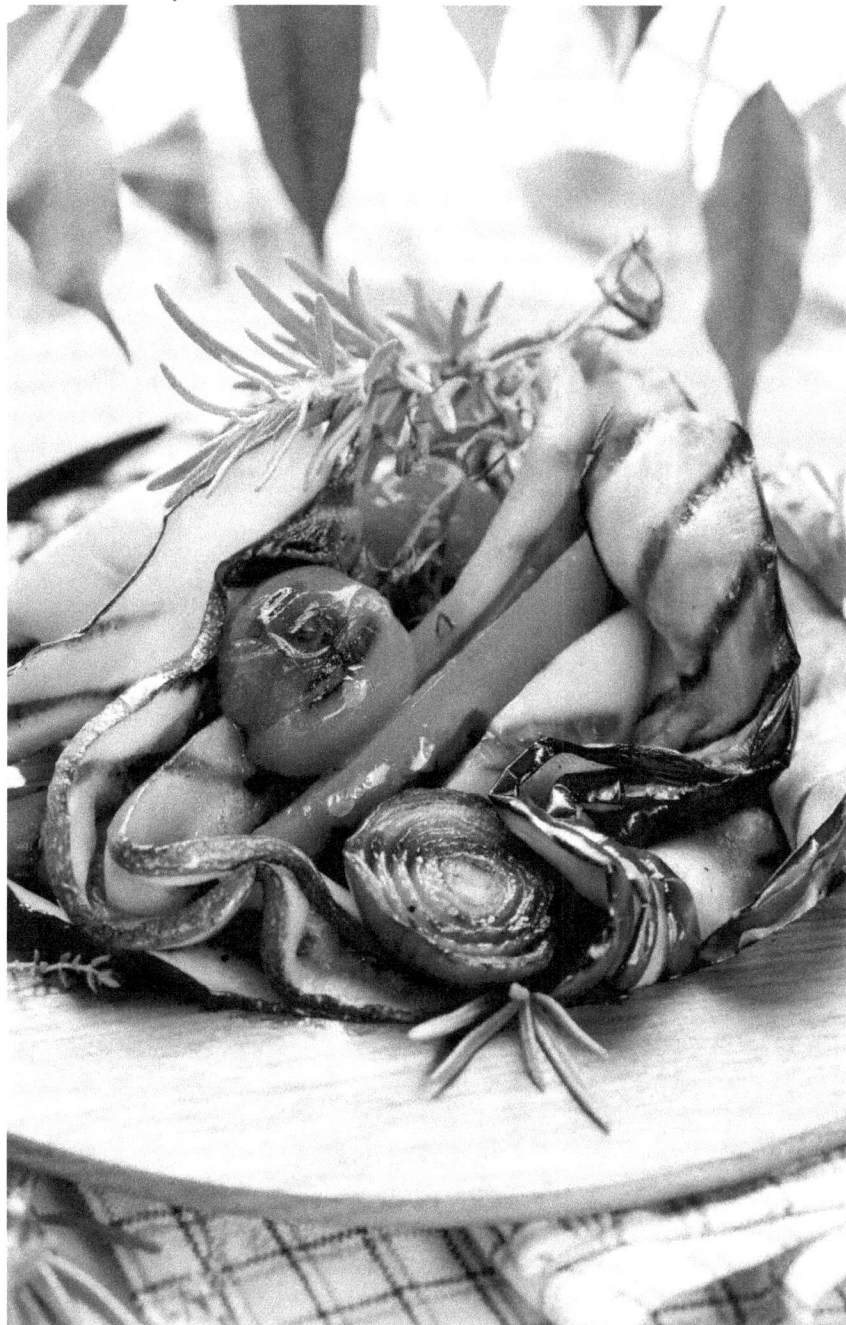

ABOUT THE AUTHOR

Dana Whyte was introduced to the Paleo diet when she became an adult and she found that it was quite beneficial. She lost the excess weight that she had gained and in addition to that she was also able to do more as she had much more energy to get it done. Her success with the diet led her to introduce other people to it. They encouraged her to write a book as she was so knowledgeable on the subject and that she did.

Dana is an advocate for healthy living and it starts with eating right.

www.ingramcontent.com/pod-product-compliance
Lightning Source LLC
Chambersburg PA
CBHW060704280326
41933CB00012B/2300